Distracting Dilemmas

To Help You Sleep

Distracting Dilemmas

To Help You Sleep

By

Imogen Macdonald

ISBN 978-1-4461-1852-8

Ditch the sheep

If, like me, you sometimes struggle to get to sleep or to get back to sleep having woken up in the middle of the night because you can't seem to turn off your own thoughts, then this little book is for you.

It is estimated that we are not alone and that as many as one in three of us at some point struggle either to get to sleep or to stay asleep long enough to wake up feeling refreshed. There are many reasons for inability to sleep, including physical causes such as medical conditions and hormonal changes as well as temporary factors or events such as jet lag, a high intake of caffeine or alcohol, or working night shifts. However it's estimated that possibly half of all insomnia cases are due to underlying psychological issues such as anxiety and stress. Of course the root of insomnia can be a cocktail of causes, but once you find yourself struggling to get to sleep or waking up during the night, anxiety about not sleeping becomes part of the problem itself.

This book is designed to help tackle lack of sleep arising mainly from anxiety and stress - the type of insomnia where you just can't get to sleep or get back to sleep because your head is full of thoughts that seem determined not to be pushed to the back of your mind. Maybe you're simply worrying about whether or not you've locked the back door and turned the oven off or maybe the anxiety keeping you awake is due to a specific incident, such as having an argument with someone that you keep replaying in your head or you are apprehensive about a presentation you have to do at work. Worse still you might find yourself struggling to sleep night after night if you are in a longer-term emotionally traumatic situation such as loosing your job, having financial worries or suffering grief through bereavement or a relationship ending. All of these situations are stressful enough without having to deal with them in a state of exhaustion because on top of everything you are going through you just cannot get your own thought processes to quiet down at night to let you sleep.

Having faced relationship breakdowns, bereavement, house moves, planning a wedding, fertility issues and redundancy, (though not all at the same time thank goodness!) I have experienced my share of waking in the middle of the night with a head full of non-sleep-compatible thoughts. There are a few real ways to help you improve your chances for a good night's rest, including reducing your intake of caffeine and alcohol, ensuring a good sleep environment and routine, not napping during the day and having a warm bath before bed. However, with the best will in the world if you've done all of the above and you still can't get to sleep or find yourself waking in the middle of the night, I know that when you've got so much going on in your head, relaxation or mind emptying exercises are not going to work any more than counting sheep will. The distracting dilemmas in this book are designed to give you something to focus on, shutting off the thoughts that stopped you sleeping in the first place. By distracting your mind and filling it with interesting, but not worrying or over-stimulating problems, you should soon find yourself falling asleep.

Please take the time to read the tips to using the dilemmas in this book, as doing so will give you the best chance for a good night's kip.

Sleep well.

Tips to using the dilemmas in this book

The dilemmas in this book are obviously not intended to give you more things to worry about than whatever it is that is keeping you awake, so I suggest that you follow these simple tips and you should find yourself drifting off in no time.

- **Don't read start the dilemmas until ready for bed.**

  It sounds obvious, but if you have already run through half of the exercises in your head then they won't necessarily work when you need them most. Just glance at a couple of dilemmas before you turn the light out and settle down to sleep, hopefully you won't need them but if you can't get to sleep or wake up in the middle of the night you should be able to remember them without having to completely wake yourself up.

- **Give yourself the chance to clear your head and fall asleep before trying a dilemma.**

  For a lot of us, the first chance we get to relax and wind down is when we actually get into bed. Please don't launch straight into one of these dilemmas but let your thoughts wander a bit, go through the day's activities and plan what you are going to do the next day, etc. Whilst all of the dilemmas in this book have been tried and tested and should distract you from whatever thoughts keep you awake or wake you up, you do need the chance to just fall asleep when you first get into bed before worrying that you aren't asleep quickly enough and launching yourself into a series of mind exercises.

- **Try not to create or fill in background details for the scenarios beyond what you are given.**

  The dilemmas in this book are designed to distract you from whatever was stopping you from sleeping and are not intended to fill your head with more things to worry about - so when presented with a scenario just go with the flow. For example, if faced with the dilemma of choosing just ten species of animal to save from extinction (dilemma number 3), don't bother yourself with why the planet is facing the destruction of all but a fraction of life as we know it. Trust me on this, introducing thoughts of catastrophic world disaster to your thought process at 3 o'clock in the morning will do nothing for your attempts at beauty sleep. Just go with the dilemma.

- **Don't over-complicate the dilemma and don't worry about the reality of your choices.**

Admittedly a few of you real hard-core insomniacs who need serious distraction might be helped by adding complex details and setting yourself harder challenges, but for most, adding provisos or rules to the dilemmas will not help you get your longed for shut-eye - it will wake you up. Taking the same example again of saving ten animals, just pick ten, not one for companionship, one for food, one to use as transport, etc. in this post-apocalypse civilisation. And don't worry about the reality of sustaining the food chain!

If you find that you really do need added levels of complication to help distract you and send you to sleep, then add them at a later stage after having tried the simple version first.

- **If it says list ten then you have to have ten.**

If a dilemma asks you to make a list – often ten of something – then you have to come up with ten. It's part of the mental distraction (that will help you to get to sleep) that you have to go beyond or trim down whatever would be your natural choice.

- **Try and keep it positive.**

If the dilemmas are personally upsetting then turn the page. Don't try the baby naming dilemma (a variation of number 1) if you are struggling to conceive and don't try the allocating money dilemma (number 12) if your money worries are severe enough to be the reason for your insomnia. Anger, anxiety and stress are all very bad for sleep, so don't try a particular dilemma if you can feel your adrenalin level rising. Focus on the positive choices you make solving these dilemmas.

- **Find the dilemmas that work for you.**

Not all dilemmas work for everyone. You may find that the subject matter of some dilemmas may not be distracting enough, for example if you have been in the same long happy relationship all your adult life, (well done), clearly the exercise to sort through past lovers (a variation of number 8) won't work for you. Other dilemmas you just might not enjoy or you may not be the sort of person who can think of which type of musical instrument each of your friends is most like (number 14).

Find the distractions that you enjoy and that work for you, remembering that the best ones are the ones you never finish because you have fallen fast asleep!

Contents

Dilemma 1

The name game

This is a basic distraction that I find works really well. All you have to do is run through the alphabet in your head, choosing a name beginning with each letter that you would happily take as a name for yourself. With each and every letter you have to pick a name that you would be prepared to live with for the rest of your life. No cheating on the difficult letters – that's in part what helps you fall asleep. You should be asleep well before Z.

I use this dilemma quite a lot and so rather than re-capping previously chosen names, I sometimes start at a different part of the alphabet. Either way there are several letters that I constantly struggle with.

Variations

If you enjoy this dilemma and it has worked in the past to help you sleep but you need variations

- **Choose a first name and a surname**

  Check each name you choose goes with your own surname or choose a first name and surname that go together. Choose a first name going through the alphabet as before and a surname (one that you have heard of, e.g. belonging to a friend or famous person) beginning with one of the letters either side.

- **Name a baby**

  Whether relevant to your own life or not, find a name for each letter that you would be genuinely happy giving to an imaginary child of yours. (Giving them joke names or just passable names will not help you get to sleep.) Either stick to boys or girls names or imagine that you are the lucky parent of twins – one of each!

- **Name a pet**

  Apply the same A-Z naming to a pet. Obviously, you need to be comfortable calling the name out in public, (unless your imaginary pet is a goldfish), but you can be more relaxed with the comedy names and puns than with the previous dilemma of naming a child. However, you still need to take the exercise seriously if you want to get to sleep.

- **Name a partner**

  I quite like the variation of choosing a name from each letter as before but for a partner, real or imaginary. I've never shared with my husband his list of alternative names and I'm pretty sure he wouldn't like many of them, but it does help me get to sleep. For an added level you can go through the alphabet choosing a name for yourself and for a partner, checking they go together.

Dilemma 2

Choose just six months

Don't bother yourself with how you have been given this global issue, (probably aliens trying to halve the size of the world's population?), but your dilemma is to choose only six months of the year. The other six months (and unfortunately anyone who has a birthday in those months) will cease to exist. This on the surface appears to be a bit of a negative dilemma, but the trick is to focus on who you are saving. Unless you have a huge number of friends and family with birthdays really spread across the year, this dilemma should be just enough to distract you out of your own thoughts and push you in the direction of sleep. If it really is too easy or too hard then obviously change the number of months you can save accordingly, but please don't make it too easy - make some sacrifices or everyone you know will be saved and you will still be awake!

Variations

If you have this down to a T you can simply reduce the number of months saved or

- **Save six star signs**

  For a twist, save six star signs instead of six calendar months. (I actually prefer this as I can save more friends and family this way – so clearly I shouldn't use it as it doesn't present as much of a dilemma!)

- **Fair weather friends?**

  If you want to add a further dimension, assume that the months you save keep their typical weather pattern. It becomes interesting if like me you have a lot of friends with winter and early spring birthdays. Who are you willing to keep for perpetual rain? Do you suddenly find yourself determined to save those distant cousins or friends you've not spoken to for years to justify saving July and August?

- **Saving dates**

  This is a very simple and quick dilemma in the same vein, but it might be too brutal for some of you to aid the sleep process. Imagine all the months of the year are divided into three rough thirds by date, i.e. 1st-10th, 11th-20th and 21st to the end of the month. You can save two of those thirds and, as with the above dilemma, all people with birthdays in the remaining third of dates will no longer be. A variation is to save just odd or even dates which can be very tricky.

- **Favourite months**

  Depending on how you are at holding information in your head without use of pen and paper, order the 12 months of the year 1st through to 12th according to how much you like them. Your choice can take into account festivals or events, weather, birthdays and anniversaries or any other factors that influence your feelings towards the different months.

- **Choose ten letters**

  This is a further variation on the main dilemma, but instead of choosing months you pick just ten letters of the alphabet. So you are saving just the people who have names beginning with those ten letters. If you want to be a bit more generous with this, the ten letters you choose can be used for first names, surnames and (at a push) nick names. You can actually cover a lot of your friends this way, but it is still going to be tricky.

  With ten letters to keep in mind this is a distraction best used if you are really awake rather than a gentler one to get you back to sleep if you are half awake in the middle of the night.

- **Twenty six letters, twenty six people**

  A difficult version of the above dilemma and one that involves holding a lot of information in your head is to save just one person for each letter of the alphabet. If you have a lot of friends and family beginning with the same letters then you're possibly going to wake yourself up rather then send yourself to sleep and maybe it's a distraction to use at the dentist rather than one to help you get some shut eye.

Dilemma 3

Saving only ten

Continuing with the jolly theme of the world as we know it coming to an end, the following dilemma is on the theme of saving just ten of a kind. Remember not to involve yourself with why the world is in this situation nor with trying to make your answers practical as the scenarios themselves clearly are not – just pick ten. They can either be your favourites OR (if different) the ones that you think should survive world as we know it destruction. If you really don't like the apocalypse concept then just imagine the classic desert island scenario whereby you are stranded on a desert island but you can take some things with you. In this case you can take quite a lot of civilisation with you to build your new world..... but only ten of one thing!

Obviously you can come up with your own topics, but here are a few to start you off. Choose just ten of the following to take on your modern day ark or be with you on your desert island

- Types of bird or animals
- Types of fruit (and do the same for vegetables)
- Types of cheese
- Flavours
- Herbs and spices
- Musical instruments
- Electrical items (yes you have electricity!)
- Television programmes
- Books
- Films
- Pieces of music
- Buildings
- Shops to do all your shopping in – food and clothes (including on-line options)

- We sites you can use
- Items of your clothing from your current wardrobe
- Colours of clothes you can wear

Variations

- **In order of preference**

  If you want to make this dilemma more complicated you can rank the items in order of preference in each of your lists. This will involve you holding more information in your head and should (if you found the exercise too easy) be more distracting and therefore more likely to get you to sleep. If you find the ordering difficult but like doing it, reduce the number of items on your list but don't drop to fewer than five or six.

  Remember these are not necessarily your favourite things, but what you would save/take with you to your new civilisation on your desert island.

- **One a year**

  To add interest to the ranking process imagine that in the first year on your island you only get the first thing on your list, with your second choice added a year later, your third a year after that, etc.

Dilemma 4

It's all about you......

This is another quite basic distraction. All you need to do is come up with a list of ten adjectives to describe yourself as though going for a job interview or placing a personal ad. In this scenario your list is all that prospective employers, dates, in-laws, etc. would see and you only get one list for all possible different audiences. You may want 'fun-loving' to be seen by potential dates, but by potential employers? One list, you have to have ten and it has to be truthful!

Variations

- **Fit for purpose**

    If you really don't like the one list for all audiences rule, a variation of course is to make different lists for different imaginary audiences – but they still all have to be accurate and each has to have ten. Your audience could be

    - prospective employers
    - prospective in-laws
    - other parents at your child's new school
    - members of a club (sporting, book group, social) that you hope to become a member of
    - new next door neighbours
    - friends of friends you are meeting at a dinner party

OR which ten (accurate) words would you like your partner to use about you when talking to friends or his/her work colleagues. OR which ten real attributes would you like to be the ones used to describe you at your own funeral?

- **Your ideal you**

  Now imagine the ten attributes you'd like to have. This can be a completely false description of you based on nothing more than how you'd ideally like to be and how you'd like other people to describe you. The dilemma, and what makes it more interesting, is that you have to list these attributes 1st to 10th in order of importance to you. Would you place 'beautiful' above 'intelligent'? Would you rather people described you as 'confident' or 'funny'?

- **Imagining your perfect partner**

  You can also apply this ranked list of attributes approach to imagining your perfect partner. Just be careful if you are in a relationship – looking at the person lying in bed next to you at 4 o'clock in the morning and realising that he/she doesn't have any of your top ten desirable attributes isn't going to get you back to sleep!

- **Gifts to a newborn child**

  You can also apply this ranked list of attributes to an imaginary child – though I would strongly advise against any comparisons with real children.

  Imagine (in the vein of Sleeping Beauty) that you are a good fairy (or wizard!) bestowing attributes on a newborn child as gifts. What ten traits would you give them, wisdom, looks, sense of humour? The dilemma is not just to pick ten adjectives, but to rank them 1st through to 10th. Would your list be different depending on whether the child was male or female?

- **Talented and gifted**

  When telling my four year old the story of Sleeping Beauty (see the above dilemma) I asked her what thing she'd give a newborn baby if she was a good fairy. I know this is a bit of a stretch for a four year old in terms of abstract thinking, but having told her the story I was secretly hoping she come up with something like 'being kind' or 'having friends'. The gift she would actually give a baby would be 'being good at swimming' which I thought was a great answer. A further variation on this dilemma is therefore to list the ten real skills or talents you would like for yourself, your child or a partner or friend? (Superhero powers are covered in dilemma 13.)

- **How you'd physically like to be**

  If you have low self esteem about how you look then this is one to avoid – it won't make you feel any better and it'll be too easy as you've probably already analysed what you think are your worst features! Clearly it won't help you get to sleep.

  The dilemma is to list the ten plastic surgeries you would have (imagining cost and health concerns not to be an issue). You have to come up with ten even if you only want a nose job.

  A variation, rather than altering your existing physical appearance, is to imagine those good fairies, (yes the ones from Sleeping Beauty who popped in before), bestowing physical attributes on you before you are born. What are the ten physical features you would most have liked to have? Be specific – 'good body and good face' or 'gorgeous all over' won't help get you to sleep. Rank them in order if you think it too easy.

- **Cheesy compliments**

  This is another variation on the above but doesn't involve any wish lists. The task is to pay yourself ten compliments – it's called cheesy compliments because you can be as cheesy as you like, (remember you never need to tell anyone else your list), but you have to be truthful. Therefore you can't say 'eyes like melting chocolate' if you have blue eyes! (You can imagine someone else is chatting you up if it helps.) So come up with ten complimentary things (OR ten physical things and ten personality traits to make it harder) about you that someone might say. The more specific you are, the more likely to get to sleep – so for example instead of 'nice hair' come up with a compliment about its colour, the cut or the way it hangs.

- **Sorting your skills**

  The next dilemma came about following another conversation with my four year old as I was explaining that she didn't need to be good at something to enjoy it (she couldn't always win at snap even though she liked playing it) and later the same day explaining that you sometimes have to do things that you don't enjoy but might be good at (mummy's tidying up).

The task is to decide on five things that you are good at and enjoy, five things you are good at but don't enjoy, five things you are not good at but enjoy nevertheless and five things that you are neither good at nor enjoy.

Dilemma 5

…..and your relationships

I have a lot of dilemmas in this category of relationships and enjoy using them to help me get to sleep, but relationships with other people are charged with a whole host of emotions, so choose which distractions you do according to your own personality and experiences. Remember these exercises are designed to help you get to sleep.

When I was made redundant I would wake up in the middle of the night really angry and I used this is dilemma to calm me down. The task I set myself was to list my ten most important relationships. These are not necessarily the people you love the most and they don't need to be good relationships, but the ones that are most dominant in your life or have the most impact. If you do it firstly for your current state and then for your whole life to date it puts things into perspective. However dominant my boss was in my thoughts (and not in a good way) during my redundancy process, he didn't even get a glance when listing the relationships that have had the most impact on my life (and I took the list up to 20). Personally, though I think that if your boss is in your list of all time important relationships that you're working too hard, I would say that it's perfectly acceptable to include pets!

Variations

In all of the following dilemmas you are asked to choose ten of something. Please try to keep to this as getting to four or five and giving up, getting bored, etc. will not get you to sleep. It's not the first few easy answers that distract you out of your thoughts and into dream-land, it's those last few tricky ones.

- **Ten friendships**

  An extension of the above dilemma is to actually limit yourself to just ten friendships beyond close family. You can assume that you still have passing acquaintances with everybody else, (so the dilemma doesn't mean that you can't chat to the other parents at the school gates or pass the time of day with someone in a shop), but you only have ten people you can ring up for a chat, email, invite round to your house, be friends with on social networking sites, socialise with, etc.

- ## How we met

  Thinking through how you met each of your friends and partners chronologically running through your life is another great way to fall asleep. Though in itself more of a memory exercise, the dilemma twist can be added by ranking in order the friends you met in the most unusual way, or the most open to chance of it not happening. (For example, I have a close friend that I met by being sat next to her on a plane, so she would be quite high ranking in my list of unusual ways I met my friends.)

- ## Perfect friends

  It's always good to know a plumber/doctor/lawyer. For this dilemma, simply choose the ten professions you'd like your friends to have between them…….. on the understanding of course that they don't charge for their services and are willing for you to ring them day or night for advice/house calls.

  For the sake or your sleep, you can make two lists – one with real jobs and one where you don't need to know the actual job titles, or even if the role really exists, for example 'wine and chocolate market researcher with lots of free samples' or 'person who has to take models out to dinner and gets to bring a friend' will sort of do. But try the real list first.

- ## Best friends

  Handle this one carefully and keep the results to yourself! Quickly think of a few superlatives (prettiest, cleverest, happiest, kindest, etc.) and then choose which of your friends fits each bill. To make it harder each friend can only be the best or most of one thing. Keep all of the qualities positive – working out which of your acquaintances has the worst dress sense or is the meanest with money might seem like fun at 4 o'clock in the morning but won't help you sleep and could sour an otherwise perfectly good relationship.

  To make it harder, you can also limit your selection pool – for example just choose from people you were at school with, work colleagues or the parents of your children's friends.

- **Who could you live with**

  Sticking with real not imaginary friends for this dilemma. Very simply choose ten friends that you could share a house with (though not all at the same time). On the surface this seems a quick dilemma, but even the most easy-going of us might not want to live with close friends if we really think about it. You can't choose anyone you currently share with - so no children, partners or current flat mates can be listed.

- **Who could you holiday with**

  An easier variation of the above dilemma is to choose ten people you could go on holiday with. Remember the first few might be easy but you have to keep going to ten – imagining just the two of you alone for two whole weeks!

- **Choose ten people to sack**

  Depending on the size of the place you work, choose just ten people you'd like to work with or if you can handle it without the 'power' waking you up, choose ten people to sack.

  ……….And finally changing tack slightly

- **Bring ten people back from the dead**

  Personally I rarely use this dilemma as I get too emotionally involved and it wakes me up (and wakes up my poor husband who finds me sobbing apparently for no reason next to him in bed at 4 o'clock in the morning). However if you are made of sterner stuff than I am, then imagine that you can bring back ten people from the dead. These can be people you knew and loved (hence the sobbing), strangers you have heard or read about and feel deserve to have lived longer or famous people. And yes, if you really must, you can have pets in this list too.

  A milder variation (which I can subscribe to) is to choose ten fictional characters that died during the course of a book/film/TV programme that you would grant a longer existence to. You can choose between allowing the characters to live on in their fictional worlds (which might destroy or improve the rest of the story) or allow them to live in an imaginary elsewhere thereby saving them but not altering the plot in the original book/film.

Dilemma 6

A friend in need

Arguably this dilemma could neatly fit into the previous one after you've selected your ten friends for life, but it's one I use quite a bit and feel justified in giving it its own place.

In this dilemma you are the friend in need in the title. Give yourself a series of scenarios and choose just five people you know to help you. They don't necessarily need to be your closest buddies but they must be more than passing acquaintances. So who would you choose to be with you if you were

- Stranded on a desert island
- In charge of running the country
- In charge of writing a Sunday newspaper (and all the different sections)
- Putting together a general knowledge quiz team to win a £1 million prize
- Putting on a show
- Going on trial and needed a good defence team
- Trying to escape from prison
- Training for the marathon
- Managing a shop

You get the idea. Make sure you try and quickly think of a scenario before you think through your friends.

Variations

- **Godparents or good parents**

  And on a slightly different note which five people would you trust to raise your children? (Don't fill in background details and imagine that you're dead – thinking about your orphaned children won't help you to get to sleep.) OR if that is too distressing, which five people would you be willing to donate your eggs/sperm to? OR which five people would you put in charge of your children's education and teaching them all they need to know?

For all of the above dilemmas you can add variety by limiting the group of people you choose your five helpers from so that you are just picking from work colleagues or family or famous people, (breaking the rule, for most of us at least, of choosing just people we know), or a specific group of well known people such as actors, musicians, etc. Just remember you are picking people you think can help you in the scenario – not the five famous actors you would most like to be stranded on a desert island with!

Dilemma 7

Sporting chance

The problem with some sporting dilemmas is that if you are really passionate about your sport then certain exercises can wake you up rather than send you to sleep. Creating your own fantasy football (or other sporting) team is a great dilemma, but if you use this to get to sleep then you may want to miss out the detail of how much each player costs and what budget you have. This invariably would need paper and pen and lists of current prices – none of which helps with the insomnia.

But the basic dilemma of selecting the best team possible should be distracting enough to take your mind off what is stopping you sleep. Variations, for those of you who haven't already thought of them, include making your team up entirely of UK players or international players, dead or retired players, those with names in the first half of the alphabet (up to M) or second and depending on the level of your knowledge, only from northern clubs or counties, those who have never competed in a world cup or equivalent in their sport, etc. You can create your own selection criteria as long as you have the knowledge already in your head and don't need pen and paper to create your fantasy team.

Variations

- **Fantasy Olympics**

  For this dilemma you need to imagine that you are on the Olympic organising committee and (let's say due to budget cuts) you have decided that the next Games will include only ten sports. You can either just choose your ten favourite sports (and they don't necessarily need to be existing Olympic events) OR mix it up a bit and try and get a good variety for the watching public. It obviously makes it harder if you try and take the events from the winter Olympics into account too.

If you want to add levels of complexity you can try to come up with ten sports that would give all of the existing athletes an area to compete in even if not exactly their current field.

- ## A new decathlon

The variation can be twisted further whereby you imagine that a new type of decathlon is born out of these ten sports with all athletes competing in all ten events. This twist might make you re-consider your initial list of ten sports to ensure that you are really testing all areas of sporting ability of the athletes competing to become the new supreme Olympiad.

A further dilemma (depending on your sporting knowledge) is to put together a fantasy team of ten GB athletes who have the best overall chance of bringing home team or individual medals in this new decathlon style Games. You can choose to do it just from existing athletes or to also include those retired or dead who you would want in your team. OR of course you can just choose ten world athletes who you would like to see competing in your new decathlon and again this can be either a list of current sportsmen and women or all time athletes regardless of current competing (or living!) status.

- ## Sport is dead – long live sport

Olympics aside, another dilemma along the same lines is to return to the theme of saving just ten. Your task is to choose just ten sports to survive (imagining if you like that the aliens taking over the planet have banned on pain of death anyone watching or competing in any sports other than the ten you choose). Your choice can be based on what you think are the ten most worthy spectator sports to save OR the sports you'd still like to be able to participate in once the aliens rule Earth!

Dilemma 8

Match making

This is a slightly different type of dilemma in that it involves matching rather than list making and it's another of my favourites! You need to choose about eight people you know - I tend to choose four couples, though singles or a mix of couples and singles works just as well if not better. Any more than eight and you'll start to need pen and paper which of course is no use if you are trying to fall asleep. Quite simply you pair everyone off with who you think they are most compatible with as long as it's not an existing partner. All eight must be paired off so you may end up with some compromises to make the whole group work.

The trick is to choose the eight individuals or four couples really quickly to start with before thinking of the possible matches and so it helps to have the right combination of gender/sexual orientation mix (though of course when pairing people up you can choose any matches you feel would work!).

Variations

If (like me) interfering in the love lives of others helps distract you from whatever was stopping you sleep then the following variations might appeal to you.

- **Cupid at work**

  Match up your work colleagues with one another going through them one by one choosing the best match from the rest of the organisation.

- **Your friends won't thank you**

  Run through each of your friends choosing another friend's partner OR a famous person for each of them.

- **Personal cupid**

  Add yourself (and partner if you have one) into the original dilemma of match making eight people - if you haven't already done so.

If you want to focus on your own love life there are some dilemmas listed below, but be careful about what keeps you awake as this isn't about re-hashing old relationships in your head – an activity guaranteed to halt any chance of sleep.

- **The good, the bad (and the ugly)**

  Mentally list your past relationships so that you know what you define as a relationship and have a total. Then go back through them - keeping half (in that they will still have happened) and loosing half (just wiping that slate clean of them). You might find that it's not always the nice ones you want to keep!

  OR have something nice happen to half of them, such as a small lottery win maybe (nothing too good, they are ex's after all) and something bad happen to the other half (nothing extreme – plane delayed by 24 hours is the sort of thing). Even if you're not bothered either way you have to choose so that you have a 50/50 list at the end.

- **The old chestnut**

  In this dilemma, you get to choose five famous people to have sex with guilt free, even if you (or they) are in relationships it's somehow allowed. A variation of this is to list five dead people you get to have sex with (imagining of course that they are not dead!).

- **The ones that got away**

  Choose ten people from your past that you would have liked to date. You have to come up with ten even if you haven't got any regrets or lost loves - remember the harder it is the more likely you are to fall asleep.

Dilemma 9

Famous friends

This is another of my favourite dilemmas and a very simple one whereby you cast friends or people you know into existing film or television roles. Simply pick a film with a good three or four main characters and cast people you know into those roles. They don't have to look like the existing actors – it is the character role you need to fill so treat the dilemma as though the film hasn't yet been shot and you are casting it for the first time.

The same can be done for a television programme, be it selecting the panel for a talent finding show searching for the next great pop sensation or casting you friends and family in your favourite soap. You can also think of a book you like or the current one you are reading and imagine it is going to be made into a film and you have to choose the cast.

One of the things I like about this dilemma and why I use it a lot is the fact that I can change it every night by selecting the programme or film that I have just watched. If you find you are using the same people again and again then put limitations on who you can use, for example just people you were at school with, (depending on your age the exercise of remembering your class mates might send you to sleep in itself!), your children's friends or their teachers, only people you know who live or work within your local community, only family, only work colleagues, etc. Don't make it too hard, but there's no dilemma (and no sleep) if you keep casting yourself and your partner into all the leading roles!

Variations

- **Your life as a movie**

  This variation swaps things around and has the famous people playing you and your friends. Imagine your life is being turned into a film – which famous people would you cast to play your friends and relatives? It's fun but can't be used more than a few times unless you cast different scenes from your life each time - more of a mini series with different themed episodes. For example, imagine there's a work based episode and you have to cast famous people to play all of your colleagues, or a flash back spanning your love life to date where you need to cast all of the people you've had relationships with, or a scene set at your local shops where the shop keeper and lollypop lady need to be cast.

- **Matching friends to jobs**

A simple variation is to think of some professions and match your friends to them. They don't necessarily need to be jobs belonging to famous people or famous jobs. Listed below are some suggested roles, but you should easily be able to think of some in the night without having to wake yourself up too much or turn on the light. It's harder if you only use each of your friends once and of course you can't cast anyone you know in their actual job (in case you hang out with TV presenters or the royal family).

So, who would make the best

- King or queen or playboy prince
- Prime minister or president
- Newsreader
- Stand up comedian
- Premiership footballer
- Model
- Agony aunt or therapist
- Stylist
- Children's TV presenter
- Judge

- **Matching friends to history**

Imagine that a number of famous people from the past have been reincarnated into people you know. In this dilemma you simply match friends and family to individuals from the past – again looks aren't essential (and you don't even need to match gender) it's more about matching the personality and/or talents based on your own knowledge (wide or limited) of the historical figure. Which of your friends, family or work colleagues is the reincarnation of

- Henry VIII
- Marilyn Monroe
- Einstein
- Florence Nightingale
- Columbus
- Shakespeare
- Abraham Lincoln
- Queen Victoria
- Charlie Chaplin
- Elvis
- Churchill

I've given some pretty obvious ones here, but you get the picture. If you can't think of anyone in your circle of friends and acquaintances to match to the historical figure keep trying – the tricky ones are what will distract you and get you to sleep, not the ones where you have an obvious match.

Having a particular area of knowledge (be it past scientists, athletes, US presidents, kings and queens of England, Hollywood stars from the 20th century, etc.) and running through the topic matching your own acquaintances as you go works particularly well, but each of your friends can only be the reincarnation of one of the people from your list.

As mentioned in the main dilemma, if you want to make things harder, then use only one set of people to fill all the roles, for example only family, work colleagues, people on your Christmas card list, your children's class mates, etc.

• **Famous friends for life**

As this section is called famous friends, this last dilemma is to choose ten famous people to be your friends. The down side is that they would replace your real friends (so you'll have no one to brag to that you went for a pint with David Beckham last night or that your shopping buddy is Jennifer Aniston). It's a bit like the classic interview question of who you'd invite to a dinner party, but in this scenario you're stuck with your choice for more than one evening and you have none of your real friends.

You can do further variations on this theme with people from the past, fictional characters or stick to one group of famous people – musicians, actors, politicians, sports personalities, etc.

Dilemma 10

Travel and leisure time

If you have ever listed all of the places you want travel to, then this dilemma might appeal to you and more importantly might get you off to sleep. The dilemma is to choose just ten countries that you can travel to and visit for the rest of your life. If you want to imagine a background scenario, then choose between the previously mentioned alien invasion whereby all of the countries you don't choose get destroyed, or the more friendly version whereby you have (for reasons I'll leave you to come up with) some sort of tag or visa restrictions whereby you alone can't travel to any more than your ten chosen countries. The second scenario, whilst obviously more humane, does mean that you don't have to save countries you think are important (globally or to yourself) even if you don't want to go there or have already been and don't want to go back there. Version two is therefore easier and so you might want to start with the personal visa restriction scenario and progress to the more brutal destruction of all but ten countries on the planet version!

Variations

This tourism style of dilemma can be applied to a variety of subjects

- **Choosing just ten cities**

  As with the above initial dilemma, you can opt for one of the two variations whereby either all other cities bar your ten are destroyed or the world is fine and all cities intact but you are just restricted in terms of your visitation allowance.

  You can also do this with **UK cities or counties, European countries, US states** or **world landmarks**, but in each of these cases you only get to save five (well it can't be too easy or there'd be no dilemma, no distraction and no sleep).

- **Leisure activities**

  Another variation on the above dilemma is to imagine that your social life and what you do in your free time (or your work time if you're a restaurant critic) is going to be limited to just five of any activity.

  Depending on your lifestyle and preferences (remember this has to be tricky enough to face you with a personal dilemma) come up with no more than five choices for any of the categories below for you to be limited to visiting/using for the rest of your life. This may just be a top five list for some of you but it's not necessarily about favourites, it's about what can sustain repeat visits for you when all of your other leisure and experience options have been cut off. So choose just five of the following to visit/see/use

  - Restaurants
  - Museums/galleries
  - Theatres
  - Cultural events/festivals
  - Bands to see play
  - Historic houses and buildings
  - Gardens
  - Beaches to surf, mountains to climb, slopes to ski

- **Home is where the heart is**

  In a slight twist, the world remains the same but the human population has been wiped out – all but you of course. Your dilemma is to decide where you will live. Don't worry about packs of roaming rabid dogs or the need for food, or how you would get there in the first place, you just have to choose where you physically want to live in the world. You can base your decision on climate or architecture (which remains intact in this post human world) or the desire just to be somewhere with personal memories. But you have to come up with ten places.

  If you need to make it a bit trickier, rank your ten places to live 1st through to 10th.

Dilemma 11

Time travel

Though not to be used regularly as they don't stand up to frequent repetition, these time travel dilemmas are nevertheless distracting enough to help you get to sleep once in a while.

You simply have to choose five times or specific events throughout history you would like to travel to. It's your dilemma so you can imagine going merely as an invisible and safe observer or as a 'hands-on traveller' spending time living the lifestyle! Your list may be different depending which you choose.

Variations

- **Living in the past**

    A simple variation on the initial historic time travel theme is to choose a time (and place) when you would actually like to live. Imagine that you are going to be sent back in time with no way of returning to the present. You can assume that somehow you'll have enough money to see you comfortably off and will miraculously talk like those around you and fit in, but you will have to make a new life for yourself. The dilemma can be split into two - picking a decade within the last (20th) century and a time prior to that.

    OR you can pick a year to be born in so that you live through different decades at different ages (though this really works only for the 20th century unless you have a good knowledge of history).

- **A life in the past**

    In a slight twist on the above, your dilemma is to choose someone whose life you would have liked to lead. So you are choosing not just the time to live but a specific life to live. Again you can split this into two dilemmas - choosing someone from the 20th century (and of course they don't necessarily need to be dead yet!) and someone from before that.

- ## A fictional life

  If you still aren't asleep then a further variation is to think of a fictional character (book, film, play, TV programme) whose life you would like to live. But it's not just a taster, you get the full life that we the audience/reader knows about.... You can't just be Cinderella after she's met her prince, you've got the loss of a mother and the years of hardship and sleeping in cinders thrown in too.

  A twist is to pick a particular group of fictional characters (fairy tale princesses, chick flick heroines, film gangsters, TV detectives, etc.) and list in order of preference the five characters whose lives you would like to lead.

- ## Personal time travel

  The personal version of this dilemma needs to be handled with care and you may find it too emotive and not conducive to sleep depending on your nature and the choices you make. In this dilemma you have to choose five times from your past to re-visit. You can go as an observer, merely to re-experience and bottle the memory or go back to change things or put them right.

  Neither version of this personal dilemma work for me as I find myself far too involved. I either want to go back to spend happy times with now dead loved ones (and sobbing into my pillow doesn't help anyone get to sleep) or I imagine myself going back in time and having conversations with past lovers or bosses and telling them what for! Regret and anger do not make happy bed fellows (any more than sorrow does), but if you can stay just a little a bit more detached than I can, then give this dilemma a go.

Dilemma 12

Who wants to be a millionaire?

This was a favourite of my Grandma's. Years ago, my lovely Grandma, on waking in the wee hours, would divvy up an imaginary million, spending on herself and giving away varying amounts.

The trick to making this work is to split the money across enough friends and family/objects of desire, to make the dilemma last long enough to help you to fall asleep but not to make it so complex as to need a calculator. Choose a sum that's personally large enough for you to make the dilemma interesting but not so huge as to just be a 'retire and travel the world' solution.

Variations

If you enjoy this dilemma but find it a bit too easy after one or two sleepless nights

- **Buying houses**

  If you haven't already done this as part of the initial dilemma, list ten places (in order of where you'll spend the most time) where you'd like to have a house. You have to come up with ten on the understanding that you'll spend at least some time in each during the year as you live your millionaire's life.

- **Indulgencies**

  If you haven't already done so, think of the specific luxuries or indulgencies that you can afford now that you are super rich. One of mine, for example, would be to have my bed made up with clean crisp sheets every night. Obviously I have to turn a blind eye the environmental impact of washing my sheets daily and also assume I already have a housekeeper in my rich world who would do all the bed making and sheet washing (well if I was doing it myself it wouldn't really be such a luxury). So ignoring practicalities and/or morals, what ten specific luxuries would you include in your millionaire's world.

- **Charitable fund**

  If you haven't done so already, add a 'charitable fund' to your pot or imagine that your whole 'million' has to go to charity. Choose ten charities to give your money to but note that they don't all need to get the same amount. The little bit of running addition in your head to get to your total from your ten generous donations will add to the distraction and the likelihood of sleep as the reward for your charitable thoughts!

- **Pay back time**

  Select ten individuals from your life - past or present but not close family or friends - to give an anonymous fixed sum (say £10,000) to. These could be people you felt you did a wrong to or those who showed you kindness in the past or people whose stories you have been touched by. The more obscure the better, but it must be ten.

- **Specific gifts**

  Be more specific in how you would spend your money. List ten things for each that you would buy for your partner, children, best friend, parents.

Dilemma 13

King for a day

One of the reasons why I wake in the night with thoughts spinning round my head is that I am a very organised (and yes controlling) person. I make lists and I like to manage my environment. If I can't control what's going on in my life, usually because I've got a ridiculously long to do list, then I wake up in the middle of the night. Insomnia and the anxiety behind a lot if it is for many of us rooted in lack of control.

This dilemma won't sort out what's going on in your life that's keeping you awake, but it might appeal to the control freaks among you out there who would like the ultimate management role. The dilemma is to imagine that you are King, Queen or Prime Minister and you need to come up with ten new laws or taxes. However, don't take this too seriously – the more obscure the better - and of course don't go into too much depth about the practicalities of your new laws - in this dilemma you rule a non-democratic state.

I'll give you one of my own, just to get it into print (well I told you I'm controlling!). If I was prime minister I would introduce a Christmas tax whereby anyone making money from Christmas goods before November would pay a tax. This would be on a sliding scale, with a higher percentage tax in August, reducing in September and further in October until there was no tax on Christmas shopping from November 1st onwards. Charities would be exempt which would allow people who really like to shop early to buy everything from them. The big retailers putting up Christmas decorations before any of us have had our summer holidays could still do so, but they would be highly taxed on any sales. I think it's an excellent plan.

Your new laws don't have to be quite so detailed (nothing that requires you to turn on a light and reach for pen and paper), it's more important that you get ten (though of course hopefully you'll be asleep long before then). Don't wind yourself up, this isn't about venting all your frustrations in the middle of the night, so don't try this one if you've recently been the victim of crime or have just had a tax bill. Remember you must have ten.

Variations

If you found yourself getting wound up by the previous dilemma, the more positive slant to the next one might be more to your taste.

- **Superhero for a day**

Continuing the theme of power and control, a simple dilemma (though not one to use too often as your answers may be the same each time) is to list the superhero powers you'd like to have, (for good not evil!).

You have to come up with ten in order of preference, but these powers wouldn't be cumulative, you only to get to have them one at a time. All other aspects of your current physical and mental abilities would stay the same which might change your choices - would being able to fly like Superman do you any good if like me you are a bit of a woos and couldn't fight the villains when you caught up with them?

A variation is of course to be the usual type of superhero whereby you are already strong, clever, attractive, etc. and then you get a super power on top! In that case flying would definitely be high up on my list .

- **Favourite things**

Continuing the positive note, come up with a list of ten favourite things. We're not talking about the big things like people or places but the tiny detail in the way that things look, smell, feel, sound or taste. Again the more obscure the better. (The feel of the pads on cats' paws? The sort of wet sound of stirring a big bowl of just cooked pasta? The specific taste of cheese and Marmite combined? The sight of tiny baby clothes hanging on a washing line?)

For your list of ten try coming up with two favourite things for each of the five senses.

Dilemma 14

What kind of animal are you?

The following dilemma won't suit everyone and if your mind just doesn't work this way then don't keep trying these more abstract exercises because you won't enjoy them and they won't help you get to sleep.

Those clever people in marketing and advertising sometimes carry out exercises like these among themselves to help develop a profile or brand around something or someone - it helps them to develop the product's 'personality'. The exercise is for you to ask yourself, 'If I was a type of animal what animal would I be'. For example I'd be a cat – to outsiders I can seem aloof and that I don't care and I can certainly use my claws if needed but to close family and friends I'm really just a big softy. Get the idea? In the middle of the night you can think of your own list, (and it can be as bizarre as you like based on your own knowledge, so anything from different metals to type of fish) but to give you some ideas, decide which type of the following you would be

- Fruit or vegetables
- Herb or spice
- Chocolate bar or sweet
- Building
- Flower /tree
- Musical instrument
- Transport or more specifically type of car
- Animal / farm yard animal /breed of dog/bird/fish/insect
- Colour or number
- Month or day of the week
- Item of clothing
- Flavour
- Planet

- Country/city
- Household appliance
- Drink or more specifically wine grape/particular beer
- Item of playground equipment

Variations

- **What planet are you on?**

  This is obviously a really easy dilemma to do for other people in your life too - your partner, your children, work colleagues, friends and relatives, etc. Either pick your topic and run through everyone you know OR choose someone and go through the different topics for them at the same time as you do yourself.

- **Know any lemons?**

  Or turned on its head a variation is that you start with the type of fruit (or animal or flower) and try to find someone to fit it. Which of your friends is most like an apple? A pear? A strawberry? You have to find someone you know to fit each – don't pass if the answer isn't obvious, the trickier the match the more likely you are to get to sleep.

- **Four birds walk into a bar**

  You can also apply a group matching process to the dilemma whereby you have to quickly list four friends/colleagues/family members and four types or bird/pieces of fruit, etc. the dilemma being to match them off. It's essential that you come up with the two lists (of four friends and four items) very quickly before you start pairing. The dilemma is to get the best matches for the whole group not just one or two pairings.

Dilemma 15

The number four is yellow

This dilemma is about matching up things that are not necessarily thought to go together. The idea is to try and match colours, feelings or noises to things that you wouldn't normally associate with having them. It's not just a pairing up exercise, you must really try to feel the link. If this is totally alien to your thought processes, and once you've tried it you really don't get it, then try a different dilemma. If you already associate each day of the week with a sound or each letter of the alphabet with a colour, then as someone with synesthesia, (the technical term for when a person involuntarily links one type of sensory stimulation with the sensation of another), though this process won't seem strange, I suggest you try associations that are not obvious or automatic to you.

- Run through the alphabet giving each letter a colour. You can't just pick a random colour, you must really think about what colour each letter feels like. OR you can do the same for numbers, days of the week or months of the year, assigning colours that each feels like. OR try giving a colour to each year or decade of your life based on how it felt. OR assign colours to your friends, countries or jobs you have had.

- Run through the months of the year or days of the week again giving each a personality or associated emotion OR give each day of the week a smell or taste.

- Try assigning sounds or the noise a particular instrument makes to the letters of the alphabet or months of the year or to different people you know or to weather types.

Dilemma 16

The taste of summer

This dilemma is similar to the previous one in that your task is to associate things that don't normally go together – in this case assigning flavours to things that aren't necessarily associated with having one.

Not long ago a well known UK crisp company ran a competition to come up with new flavours. Of course with one thing and another I never got round to sending in my no doubt winning entries, but during those few weeks the process of coming up with new flavours helped me get back to sleep on more than one occasion. The dilemma is to decide which ingredients you would use to create abstract flavours.

The ones I was going to enter into the competition were the four seasons, i.e. summer, autumn, winter and spring and a Friday flavour. Of course you can come up with flavours for months of the year or special occasions, (for example what ingredients would valentine flavour crisps have in them?) or imagine that you have to make crisps (or popcorn) for a film premier (what ingredients would Godfather or Pretty Woman crisps be made with?) or for a band or specific type of music? Be as abstract as you like. I set myself the task of using no more than five ingredients to make each flavour but if you really think your summer popcorn is just strawberries and cream flavour or Pimms and apple then that's your choice. Of course your crisps or popcorn have to actually taste good, (if it's going to win the competition and be commercially made and sold), so no putting in really rancid ingredients for comedy value.

Dilemma 17

War of the roses and tulips

Lots of the dilemmas so far have been about matching things up, this dilemma on the other hand is all about competition. All you need to do it choose a topic that you like, flowers, metals, cars etc., pick a couple of competitors from your topic group and give them something to compete over be it a race, a fight or a cake making competition. The competition doesn't need to be something that you would find your subject matter normally doing and in fact the more abstract and bizarre the activity the better as it will take more consideration on your part and you'll find it more distracting.

For example, taking flowers as our contestants and a fight as the competition - who would win between a rose and a tulip? Thinking about it a rose has thorns but overall seems a bit more delicate than a brash tulip. On the other hand a tulip doesn't have much stamina and once it's lost a couple of petals it's all but over, but maybe its more flexible stem would help it beat the rose? Remember this is about taking your mind off whatever is keeping you awake, so take your time and really consider why one competitor should win.

Once you have your winner, they can take on all challengers, and if you so choose your runners up can compete so that you eventually end up with, if we follow the flower example, the top five ranking fighting flowers.

I've given suggested lists of topics and competitions below, but this works best if you choose something that interests you and you know a little bit about for your contestants and competition. This isn't about firing you up, the scenario should be as obscure and abstract as possible, so try and avoid imagining real and possible situations (so no 'which country would win a war' thoughts) as it won't help you get to sleep (but feel free to imagine which country –not its residents- would win a beauty competition).

Possible contestants

- Flowers/trees/herbs
- Body parts
- Musical instruments
- Birds/insects
- Lucky charms (horse shoe, black cat, four leaf clover)
- Characters from fairy tales, super-heroes, Jane Austen's leading ladies, children's TV characters
- Celebrities, members of the royal family, politicians, previous kings and queens of England, US presidents
- Metals, stones, gem stones
- Countries/cities/counties/US states (don't think about the individuals in them but the personality and strengths of the actual countries)
- Fruits or vegetables
- Types of cheese
- Planets in the solar system
- Cars or modes of transport

Possible competitions

- A fight
- A cooking competition
- A race, tennis match (or other individual sporting event)
- Car chase
- Sandcastle building competition
- A beauty contest
- A dancing competition
- A debate

Variations

- ## The odder the better

   If you like thinking in a really abstract way then make your contestants (rather than the competition) more bizarre. So get colours or days of the week or months of the year competing, (e.g. would Friday win a sprint but Tuesday the marathon? Who would be the better cook out of the eight of spades and the three of diamonds?).

- ## The supreme flower champion

   You can make it more complex if you really need distracting, by judging the 'competitors' on a number of things rather than competing on a one to one level. So taking our previous example of flowers and assuming this is a topic you know a bit about, to find the supreme flower champion score each flower out of five on, for example, looks, physical stamina, scent, use to us humans, use to other animals – bees, rabbits! etc. With a total for each flower (out of 25) you should be able to rank your top five flowers. Just remember this is an exercise to get you to sleep so no pen and paper.

- ## Meet my lawyer - the rose

   If you've been working through this book then you've already given personalities to fruit and flowers, know which flower would win various competitions and have selected the supreme flower based on a number of criteria. The next dilemma is therefore just a small step – you have to decide which flower (sticking with that example) would be the best candidate for a number of different jobs. Who would be a better prime minister a rose or a daffodil? Who would make a better lawyer between a daisy and a tulip? As always pick a subject that you know something about and enjoy thinking about the qualities of, be it trees, planets, towns, trains, rivers, makes of car or pieces of music.

Dilemma 18

What's in a name?

This dilemma is simply about naming things, but unlike dilemma 1, you have to rename something that already has a name. So think of a film title and come up with three (one would be too easy) alternatives for that film. For example could 'Mary Poppins' be called 'Nanny Knows Best' 'Supercalifragilisticexpialidocious' or 'The Magical World up the Chimney'?

You must try and come up with three titles that would have as strong an impact on the success of the film thinking about the existing audience and what would appeal to them. Avoid trying to be funny (unless you are re-naming a comedy) as you have no audience to appreciate your wit and remember this is designed to help you get to sleep! Try not to just come up with alternative words with the same or similar meaning, for example renaming 'Star Wars' as 'Battling Universes' is not stretching your thought process enough to help with your insomnia. Try not to give the plot away unless it already is alluded to in the real title so replacing 'Dumbo' with 'The Flying Elephant' is not really okay.

It's harder than you think to come up with three good alternatives and should with any luck be distracting enough to send you off into a deep slumber. Try renaming

- Films
- Television Programmes
- Books
- Album or song titles
- Works of art

Variations

- ## That which we call a rose

  You can try renaming flowers, trees, birds, animals, body parts, fruit, etc. but rather than inventing your own word you have to rename using another from the same category. So if you had to find a new name for a rose would the word daffodil work or would lily be a better name? (I would skip this dilemma if you have a good knowledge of Latin or understanding of the derivatives of words as you might just find this frustratingly silly and it won't get you to sleep.)

- ## Rename your friends

  Without having to run through the alphabet (as in dilemma 1) pick a new name for each or your friends or family members that you think would really suit them.

- ## Keep the name – change the plot

  Twist the original dilemma around so that you keep the name of the film or book but have to come up with three alternative plots for the title. You need ideas that are completely unlike each other or the original (preferably of a totally different genre). Just a few thoughts in your head about will do - you're not being asked to write a screen play, just think about alternatives that would go with the name. Of course the difficulty and the distraction is to come up with three different ones.

  So for example, The Twilight Zone could be a) an animated story about cute little moths that come out at dusk, b) a romance about pensioners in a care home falling in love in their twilight years, or c) a thriller where the heroes uncover a chemical spillage which shows up due to the unusual sunsets seen in the sky around the industrial area responsible for the leak! Okay, I agree that they are pretty poor, but you get the idea. Try and do better.

Dilemma 19

Music to fall asleep to?

A lot of us have come up with our list of desert island music and when I grew up in the days of the mix tape I made compilations specifically designed for jogging, listening to while getting ready to go out, sad songs, ones to help me get to sleep, etc.

Your task is to come up with a play list of five pieces of music for a number of activities. You can do two lists if you like, one list of five that you would like to listen to and another list (if it's different) that you'd commercially package and sell as 'music to......'

- Run or exercise to
- Cook to
- Iron or do the housework to
- Make love to!
- Listen to on the morning of your wedding
- Play at a dinner party
- Dance to
- Have at your funeral
- Play to cheer you up
- Give you emotional strength
- Sing to in the shower
- Drive to
- Play on the beach or at a summer barbecue
- Fall asleep to!

You get the idea. If you find it's too easy extend the number to ten of each.

Dilemma 20

Incognito

A quick little dilemma this one. Imagine that you are on the run – let's say you're in a witness protection programme or if you prefer you can be a spy (!) just don't fill in too many details and worry too much about the background scenario.

Your dilemma is to think about things that would enable those you love to find you or know that you are alright whilst not giving the game away to the baddies.

- Where would you go in the world where your loved ones would think to look for you? It can't be as obvious as your honeymoon destination in case the other side found you, but it has to be somewhere that your loved ones might consider looking for you.

- What coded message could you use in an email/phone call that would let your loved ones know it was you but would seem innocuous to those who've got your family under surveillance?

- What question would you ask your partner/friend that only they would know the answer to in order to prove it was them on the other end of the email and not the baddies trying to track you down?

Dilemmas

For younger insomniacs

Many of the dilemmas listed over the previous pages are suitable (with a few tweaks) for younger insomniacs, but to make life easier for those of you woken in the middle of the night by a small voice calling out, "muuum, I can't sleep" I have listed them all here and added a few extras.

Obviously it should go without saying that you need to check that all is well before encouraging your child back to sleep, and often all a child needs is a cuddle and reassurance that the monster was really just part of a bad dream and is not under the bed. Giving them a mental task to do when they would have naturally fallen back to sleep is clearly not a good idea. If however they don't find it easy to drift off to sleep or back to sleep if waking in the night and their state of wakefulness is related to their own thoughts running round and round in their head and not anything more serious, then distraction can work well.

For young children

Often just getting a young child to imagine something nice (but not too exciting) will help them drift pleasantly to sleep. My four year old can be lulled easily by telling her to imagine a princess in a garden feeding a little kitten with some milk. I never need to get more descriptive than that before she is asleep (which is a good thing as at 4 o'clock in the morning I am not sure I could elaborate sufficiently). Again it is important not to over stimulate young children and wake them up further, so give them a chance to fall back to sleep on their own before challenging them to imagine something – and make sure that what you get them to picture is simple and restful (lists of what they want for Christmas or imagining exciting trips to the seaside won't necessarily work).

For young children struggling to get to sleep at the beginning of the night, making a mental list with them can help. People they know, friends they have, shops they go to, food they like, etc. counted along their fingers. They may not be able to do it on their own, but if you do it with them first, (I sometimes count ten of something on the set of little fingers in question), when you leave the room they will still be running through some of the answers in their head and this can really help them get to sleep.

For older children

Depending on the age of your child, all or some of the dilemmas below can help them get to sleep and get back to sleep if they wake in the middle of the night. Remember their responses to these dilemmas are private and so don't expect to be told (and don't ask) what they came up with as answers.

1. **Give yourself a new name.**

    All a child has to do is run through the alphabet in their head, choosing a name beginning with each letter that they would happily take as a name. This can also be done choosing a name for a pet or for older teens choosing names they'd like for a boyfriend or girlfriend (unless of course first love gone wrong is causing the insomnia and then this wouldn't be the right time to bring perfect partner names into the equation!).

2. **Ten things forever**

    The listing dilemma picking only ten of something that a child can have also works well. (I hope that I don't need to state that the background scenario of world destruction or abandonment on a desert island, as used in the adult version of this dilemma, shouldn't be mentioned unless you are sure it will add to the enjoyment of list making rather than add to the trauma of waking in the small hours from a nightmare.)

    Try only ten types of food they can eat, ten shops they can shop in, television programmes they can watch, web sites they can visit, friends they can have on social networking sites ......

3. **Ten animals to have as pets**

    Another listing dilemma is to get children to imagine the ten animals that they would like as pets. You can explain that the practicalities would be magically sorted out, unless you have a child who would like to think of the living arrangements for the ten creatures they choose in which case don't take that element away.

4. Matching friends to jobs

The dilemma of matching friends to jobs is one that can be done by most age groups (even those who haven't started working yet). The rules are that no one can have more than one job and no job can be done by more than one person. Simply get your child to run through jobs (prime minister, pop star, TV presenter, actor, footballer, fire-fighter, etc.) in their head allocating them out to friends or family or limit it to those in their class.

A easier variation for younger children is to just get them to come up with a list of five jobs they'd like to do when they grow up – one for each day of the week!

5. Matching friends to history or literature

Older children can probably manage the matching friends to famous people from history or to fictional characters. But this is tricky if they can't come up with an initial list to match to so make sure that they can rustle up a few kings and queens or past film stars before you go back to bed. In this dilemma they simply match friends and family to individuals from the past – looks aren't essential it's more about matching the personality and/or talents based on their own knowledge of the person.

6. Life as a movie or TV series

Most older children should enjoy the dilemma of casting actors to play them and their friends if their life was being turned into a film or TV series. You probably won't know half of the actors that they choose and certainly don't ask who they cast as you - you might not like the answer.

7. Famous friends for life

Again, older children should enjoy this dilemma and for those whose insomnia is caused by not currently getting on with their friends it's a great distraction. Simply get your child to pick ten famous people to be friends with.

8. Superhero powers

Depending on age and preferences of your sleepless child, get them to choose which five superheroes or fairy tale princesses they would be or which five characters from films. Older children can also rank these in order of preference.

A further variation is to choose which superhero powers they'd like to have – in preference order, choosing up to ten.

9. What animal would you like to be

If superheroes aren't their thing, another similar exercise is to get your child to imagine that they can be an animal for the day. Get them to imagine that they have this power for a week and can be a different animal each day.

10. Wish list

I don't know many children who don't enjoy making a Christmas list or thinking of all the things that they are going to have when they are grown up and think that money will be no object. On the whole I advise against this wish list as a way to gently get a child back to sleep, but you know your own children and it can work for some of them. Give them a limited number of imaginary things that they can have (or for older children who know the costs of things, an imaginary budget to spend) and say that they also have to get something for siblings or for you.

Basic Exercises

Distraction without dilemma

There are of course other ways to fall asleep without distracting your mind with a dilemma. The tasks listed below should help get you to sleep without the need to make any choices or moral decisions. They are exercises simply designed to distract you, help you relax and encourage sleep.

1. **Listen carefully**

   This is an exercise that focuses all your attention onto one of your senses. By doing so it both takes your mind off what woke you up and 'closes down' the other senses making you more likely to fall asleep. I've done this in busy city, quieter suburb and countryside settings. All have worked surprisingly well no matter how noisy or quiet I initially thought my location.

   The exercise is simply to close your eyes and to find the noise nearest to you (a clock, snoring husband! or your own heart beat) and to listen to it for a while before seeking out the next nearest noise and listening to that for a while. You must really focus, seeking out sounds you weren't aware of before the exercise and listen to each of them in turn. Whatever you do don't just think 'oh I can hear the central heating kicking in and cars near by'. It is a slow and gentle exercise and should focus you away from other night time thoughts.

2. **Lie back and relax**

   When I was little and couldn't sleep I was taught to play a game where I had to tense and then relax each part of my body in turn starting from my toes up right until the point when I had to relax my eyelids.

   There's nothing unique about this relaxation exercise and it is used not just to encourage sleep. However I find that the real trick is to go through enough body parts to make the process take quite some time and in doing so you should be asleep before you get to your eyelids! So don't just 'tense and relax legs', try and think about tensing and relaxing each toe, sole of the foot, ankle, heel, calf, knee, etc. doing so separately for each leg.

3. Dare to dream

This exercise is not for those of you who don't picture things easily in their heads nor at the other extreme for those of you who have very vivid dreams and have woken following a nightmare and have unpleasant images already in your mind.

You need to have your eyes closed and to try and see an image or picture or just colours 'in your mind's eye' and to let these images go where they want to – you mustn't control the picture. Sometimes it helps to start the process off by picturing something simple, say an apple with a butterfly landing on it, and then just try to let the image go on from there. Really focus on the image and what it is doing. Of course you aren't really starting the dream process but if you can do this exercise, you are relaxing, closing down some of your senses and hopefully all of those thoughts that woke you up in the first place.

4. A-Z

An exercise with endless variations and different levels of difficulty is a simple A-Z game. Decide on a topic and then run through the alphabet in your head coming up with something from your category beginning with each letter in turn. Good category choice is essential, if you make it too easy you'll be at Z in no time and still awake, but you do need a category of which you have some knowledge or experience. I've listed a few basic examples below, but you should be able to come up with some interesting categories of your own depending on personal knowledge and preference.

- Flowers/trees/fruits/vegetables
- Famous people (you can use a category of fame, so actors/writers/singers/athletes, etc. or restrict yourself to just first or last names)
- Fictional characters
- Bands or song titles
- Item of clothing
- Countries/towns/cities

- Animals/birds/insects
- Cars (makes and/or models)
- Gem stones/precious metals
- Rivers, seas and lakes

5. Sex it up

This is not nearly as exciting as it sounds but I make no apologies as excitement and sleep do not go hand in hand. The exercise is simply to give a male/female label to non gender specific items. This might not work for you if you are a linguist or indeed can speak any language which applies a gender to nouns and so already have a male/female view of items.

You can simply look round your dark room or at the bedside table and if you can give a male or female label to each piece of furniture or item then close your eyes, relax and run through the days of the week, numbers, countries, colours, fruit, furniture, clothing etc. applying a gender to each. A variation is to apply a gender to verbs, emotions, memories, years of your life, etc.

6. No cutting corners

This is a simple counting exercise and though it involves no sheep it does involve a bit of visualisation and concentration which is why it works as a distraction. Go through the alphabet picturing the letters in capitals counting the number of corners or intersections on each letter. It is easier and gives you more corners if you imagine them as outlines or really thick chunky letters. So a simple outlined capital H (without any serifs or fancy little feet) would give you a count of 12. You can simply go through the alphabet (or through numbers) counting the intersections or for a bit of variety compare the names of friends seeing whose name has the most corners.

If you like this version of a counting exercise and it works for you then you are in luck as the variations should keep you going night after night! You can simply choose a category (e.g. fruit) and compare say apples and bananas or you can try and find the fruit with the most (or least) number of corners when written in chunky capitals.

7. Valuing your friends

Another simple counting exercise is to assign a number to each letter of the alphabet, A=1, B=2, etc. through to Z=26. You simply add up the value of all of the letters in your first name to come to a total. Run through your friends and find the person with the lowest value name or the highest, can you beat my friend Kathryn whose name though starting with a relatively low K (with a value of 11) manages to fit a Y in there and gives her a high score of 97! Of course you can apply this counting exercise to other topics and rank trees, fruit, places, etc.

8.   Homework

This is a simple visualisation exercise whereby you imagine in turn each room in your house. Choose one of the categories below and as you picture each room list all of the objects that fit into your selected category. I have come up with a few examples

- All electrical items (and all items with batteries)
- All circular or square shaped objects
- Everything that begins with A (or B or C or D.......)
- Everything the colour blue, or brown, or black, etc.

9.   Count your encounters

This is a memory exercise whereby you start as far back as you can remember and simply run through everyone you've ever known. Try and remember their names but don't worry if you can't – it's just a list for you so 'the lollypop lady by primary school' is okay as long as you really remember her and are not just making it up because you assume there was one. Try and dig deep and recall anyone you can – neighbours, people you met on holiday, old play friends, people from your first job.

10. Letters be friends

Run through the alphabet in your head counting how many people you know whose names begin with each letter (you can weight the results if you like giving more points for a good friend or close family member). Do certain letters get a much higher score for you? Is there a pattern? Can you spell anything out with those letters? Do they all fall in a certain part of the alphabet?

An ex boyfriend of mine has never had a girlfriend with a name in the second half of the alphabet (not intentionally) and I have a far higher number of friends whose names start with one of the letters in my name than with any other letters (again not intentionally and something I've only just noticed). Try and find a pattern for the letters that seem key in your life even if there isn't an obvious one there.

Final thoughts

Not all of the dilemmas will have worked for you and you may enjoy some more than others, but I hope this little book has helped you get to sleep or back to sleep when you need it most. If you've developed your own variations of the dilemmas in this book or come up with new ones, remember to keep a note of them (I've conveniently left some space for you below) so that you have them when you need them most.

Sleep tight.

www.ingramcontent.com/pod-product-compliance
Lightning Source LLC
Chambersburg PA
CBHW060644290526
45793CB00001B/390